Everyday DASH Diet Recipes

50 Delicious Recipes to Promote Weight Loss, Prevent Diabetes, Lower Cholesterol and Relieve Hypertension.

Table of Contents

About the Book

This recipe book has been written with the DASH Diet in mind and is meant to provide you with healthy, delicious, and easy recipes that you need in order to follow this diet plan. The DASH Diet provides you with a way to enjoy great tasting foods while keeping you within the required dietary guidelines and allowing you to live a healthier life.

The DASH Diet a great way to start a healthy new lifestyle for anyone who wants to lose weight, lower high blood pressure, and feel and look better. These recipes are full of the fruits, vegetables, vitamins and minerals that your body needs to live a healthy life without taking out any of the taste. Take a little time to search through these recipes and find your new favorite recipe of the day!

Introduction

The DASH Diet is a great way to receive many of the vitamins, minerals, and other nutrients that your body needs in order to stay healthy and feel great. This diet plan does not limit the amount and types of food that you enjoy while following it; in fact, it encourages a wide variety of fruits, vegetables, whole grains, meats, and dairy products for you to enjoy.

Chapter 1 starts out with some yummy breakfasts that you are sure to enjoy with your whole family. From pancakes to fruit and everything in between you are sure to find something that everyone will enjoy. Chapter 2 dives into some delicious salads that you can either add as a side to your main meal or enjoy them as their own meal.

Chapter 3 introduces you to some new soup ideas that are great if you are looking for a little something to fill you up without all the extra calories. You can enjoy Minestrone Soup or even a fun Shamrock soup throughout your day. Chapter 4 shows you some of the unique sides to your main course that you are sure to love.

Chapter 5 is a precursor to the main dishes by giving you a little taste of Italy in the form of some great pasta; whenever you are looking for something simple to make for your family that will fill them up, make one of these quick pasta ideas that they will love. Chapter 6 is the main event and provides you with a wide variety of main dishes to make for lunch and for supper.

Follow these delicious meals with some decadent desserts in Chapter 7. These desserts will make you feel like you are cheating on your diet each time you enjoy them.

Chapter 1 –Breakfasts Galore

Ricotta Pancakes with Orange and Raspberries

4 eggs
2 Tbsp. sugar
1 /13 c. ricotta cheese
1 Tbsp. orange rind
2 Tbsp. butter
1 c raspberries
½ c. flour
Maple syrup
Salt

Start out by mixing together the orange rind, sugar, ricotta, and egg yolks until they are creamy before adding in the salt and the flour. In another bowl you will beat the egg whites into stiff peaks and then whisk the egg whites with the ricotta mixture. You can then spoon all of the batter onto a griddle until small bubbles show up on the pancakes and then flip them over and cook the other side. Serve the pancakes with syrup and raspberries.

Feta Cheese, Mushroom, and Spinach Scramble

½ c. mushrooms
1 egg
2 egg whites
1 c. spinach
1 Tbsp. feta cheese
Pepper

Heat up a sauté pan and spray on some cooking spray before adding the spinach and the mushrooms. Sauté the spinach and the mushrooms for about 3 minutes; the spinach should be wilted. Next you will whisk together both the egg whites and the eggs in a small bowl along with the feta cheese. Pour this mixture over the spinach and mushrooms and continue to cook the whole mixture for another 4 minutes until the eggs are cooked all the way through.

Overnight Oatmeal

4 cups of milk
2 cups oats
½ c. raisins
4 cups of water
1/3 c. dried cherries
1 tsp. molasses
1/3 c, dried apricots
1 tsp. cinnamon

Put the milk, oats, raisins, water, dried cherries, dried apricots, molasses, and cinnamon in the slow cooker and turn the heat on low. Stir the ingredients together so that they can set and then turn the heat on low. Cover with the lit and let it cook for at least 8 hours. When it is ready spoon the oatmeal into bowls and then serve.

Frittata

6 eggs
1 c. pepper strips
1 c. grape tomatoes
1 c. sweet corn
¼ c. onion sliced
4 oz. cheese blend
2 Tbsp. canola oil
1 tsp. basil

Stir together the eggs and then add some basil before setting this mixture to the side. Pour some canola oil onto a frying pan and then add the sweet corn, onion, and pepper strips and sauté for about 3 minutes. Next you will need to add the tomatoes and stir for another 5 minutes. Pour the mixed eggs over these vegetables and then using a spatula lift up the edge to allow the eggs to end up at the bottom as it cooks. You can top the frittata with cheese once the egg is thick. Cook for another 3 minutes before serving.

Very Berry Museli

1 c. oats
1 cup yogurt
¼ c. walnuts
½ c. milk
½ c. apple, chopped
½ c. mixture dry fruit
½ c. blueberries frozen
Salt

Mix together the salt, milk, yogurt, and oats in a bowl before covering and letting it set in the refrigerator for around 6 to 12 hours. Once the time has passed you can add on all of the fruit, the fresh and the dried and mix in gently. Serve in small bowls and sprinkle with the walnuts. Do not leave the mixture out for more than 3 hours.

Fruit and Gain Salad

3 c. water
¾ c. brown rice
¾ c. bulgur
1 orange
1 apple; Granny Smith
1 apple, Red Delicious
1 c. raisins
8 oz. yogurt
Salt

Bring some water and the salt to boiling in a large pot. Once the water is bowling you can add in the bulgur and the rice and cook for about 10 minutes on reduced heat and covered. After that has cooked you can take off the heat and set aside for about 2 minutes. Spread out the grain on a baking sheet and let them cool; you can do this step the night before just make sure to keep them in the refrigerator after cooling. Right before you are ready to serve you will prepare the fruit by chopping the apples and cutting the orange. Move the grains and fruit to a mixing bowl and add in the yogurt until everything is coated.

No Bake Granola Bars

2 ½ c. rice cereal
½ c. raisins
1 c. oatmeal
½ c. brown sugar
½ c. corn syrup
½ c. peanut butter
1 tsp. vanilla

Combine together the raisins, oatmeal, and rice cereal in a bowl and stir together. In a saucepan you will need to mix together the corn syrup and the brown sugar. Stir constantly until the mixture is boiling; remove the saucepan right away once the mixture is boiling. Stir in the vanilla and peanut butter and blend until the mixture is smooth. Pour this mixture over the raisins and cereal in the bowl and mix it all together. Put this whole mixture into a baking pan and let it cool.

Banana Nut Pancakes

1 c. flour, whole wheat
2 tsp. baking powder
1 banana
1 c milk
2 tsp. oil
2 Tbsp. walnuts
1 tsp. vanilla
Salt
Cinnamon

Mix the flour, baking powder, banana, salt and cinnamon in one bowl while combining the bananas, vanilla, egg white, and milk in another bowl before adding both of the bowls together and mixing until it is all a liquid. Heat a skillet and spray it with cooking spray. Pour about ¼ of this batter for each pancake and once the batter is bubbling on one side you can flip the pancake over and cook the other side.

Bread Pudding

1 ½ c. milk
4 eggs
½ tsp. vanilla
2 Tbsp. brown sugar
½ tsp. cinnamon
4 slices wheat bread
¼ c raisins
½ c. apple
2 tsp. sugar; powdered
Salt

Start this recipe by preheating the oven to about 350 degrees. While that is heating up you can combine the salt, cinnamon, vanilla, brown sugar, eggs, and milk. Mix all together until well combined. Add the raisins, apple, and bread and mix again until combined and the bread cubes are soaked. Transfer this mixture to a baking pan and bake for about 40 minutes while covered with foil and then uncover and bake for another 20 minutes. Let the pudding set and cool for around 10 minutes before serving.

Chapter 2 –Leafy Greens

Tuna Plate Salad

1 can tuna
1 egg, hard-boiled
2 Tbsp. mayonnaise
¼ c. celery
1 c. lettuce, romaine
Pepper strips
Red cabbage
Grape tomatoes
Grated carrots

Mix the mayonnaise, celery, egg, and tuna together in a big bowl. Next you will make a base for the salad with the romaine lettuce and top it with any sliced vegetables that you would like. Place some of the tuna on top of it all and enjoy.

Apple and Pistachio Salad

1 c. yogurt
3 apples; Granny Smith
1/3 c. pistachios
¼ tsp. cayenne pepper
1/3 c. blue cheese
Pepper
Lemon juice

Mix together the yogurt and the pepper and place to the side. Next you will need to core and cut up the apple and squeeze some of the lemon juice on them before tossing in with the pre-made yogurt mixture. Let this all cool in the refrigerator for about an hour. Right before you are ready to serve the salad you should add the pistachios and blue cheese to the apple mixture and mix it all together.

Blueberry, White, and Red Salad

2 c. cubed watermelon
2 Tbsp. lemon juice
2 oz. feta cheese
1 c. blueberries
1 Tbsp. mint leaves

Start by combining the lemon juice, blueberries, and watermelon and mix them until they are mixed together. Chill these fruits until it is time to serve them. Right before you are ready to serve the salad you should add the mint and the feta and toss together until they combined.

Carrot and Dried Plum Salad

2 lbs. carrots
¼ c. lemon juice
½ tsp. paprika
¼ cumin; ground
2 Tbsp. olive oil
1 c. plums
2 Tbsp. sesame seeds
3 Tbsp. cilantro
Salt

Cut up the carrots into pieces that are about 1 inch pieces. Put the carrots into some boiling water and cook for around 5 minutes until they are tender but you do not want them to become mushy. Drain them and rinse them off right away with cold water and set aside. Next you can mix the salt, cumin, paprika, oil, and lemon juice together in a bowl before adding in the cilantro, plums, and carrots and mix together. Place the salad on the plates to serve and sprinkle with some sesame seeds.

Corn and Black Bean Salsa Salad

1/3 c. olive oil
1 garlic clove
Cumin
Coriander
¼ lime juice
2 c. black beans
2 c. corn
2 jalapeno chilies
¾ c red pepper
¾ c. orange pepper
¾ c. onion
½ c. cilantro
1 tomato

Start by making the dressing. Whisk the coriander, cumin, garlic, lime juice, and olive oil together until it is blended. Let this set aside for about 30 minutes to allow it to blend. While that is setting you can combine the onion, jalapenos, bell peppers, corn, and black beans together. Pour the dress that you already made on the salad and toss it all together to combine. Lastly you will add in tomato and toss a little more. Let this salad chill for a couple of hours before serving. Add the parsley and toss well before serving.

Chapter 3 –Hearty Soups

Minestrone Soup

¼ c. olive oil
1 carrot
1 celery stalk
1 onion
2 potatoes
1 c. tomatoes, chopped
1 c. cannellini beans
1 kale bunch
½ c. parmesan cheese

Start by heating up the olive oil in a large pot before adding in the celery, carrot, and onion. Make sure to sprinkle this mixture with a little bit of pepper and salt to taste. Let this cook for around 15 minutes until the vegetables are soft. Next you can add in the potatoes and let cook for another 10 minutes before adding in about 6 cups of water and stir it around making sure to remove all brown bits on the bottom. After adding the tomatoes you can bring the water to a boil and then let it simmer for another 15 minutes. Finally you will add the kale and zucchini and then increase the heat to steady bubbling. Cook for about 15 more minutes before stirring in the beans and cooking for another 4 minutes. Top the soup off with some olive oil and cheese to taste.

Shamrock Soup

½ c. celery
½ c. onion
½ c. carrot
¾ c. split peas
1 can of chicken broth
1 ½ c milk
1 Tbsp. butter
4 c. spinach leaves
Salt
Pepper
Nutmeg

Start by sautéing the celery, carrot and onion in the butter until soft. Then you should add half milk, chicken broth, and the split peas. Bring all of this to a boil and then let simmer for about 30 minutes, making sure to stir it until the peas feel tender. Take the mixture off the heat and let it cool down. Once that is cooled you should puree to spinach with this pea mixture. Return it all to the saucepan and stir in a little more milk. Cook until the mixture is simmering and then season with nutmeg and pepper to taste.

Spicy Chili

2 Tbsp. olive oil
1 lb. chicken breast
1 Tbsp. garlic
1 pepper
2 carrots
1 onion
1/3 c. chili powder
1 onion
15 oz. kidney beans
2 cans diced tomatoes
2 cans beef broth
Pepper salt

In a pot sauté up the chicken breast with olive oil until the chicken is browned on each side and then remove the chicken to set aside. In that pot combine the carrots, bell peppers, and garlic together and sauté until brown for about 5 minutes before adding in the chili powder and sautéing for about 3 more minutes. Finally you will need to add in the cooked chicken, broth, tomatoes, and kidney beans. You will need to simmer this liquid for about 15 minutes. Add in any pepper and salt if you want to.

Beef Soup

1 lb. ground beef
1 carrot
2 garlic cloves
1 celery
1 onion
8 c. water
1 c. barley
14.5 oz. diced tomatoes
1 cube beef bouillon
Pepper

Cook up the ground beef in a skillet before adding garlic, celery, onion, and carrots and stir them all around for 5 minutes. Next you should add the barley, tomatoes, bouillon, and the water, reduce the heat and then let it all cook for up to 40 minutes. You can add some pepper to taste after it is cooked and serve right away.

Tomato, Corn, and Acorn Squash Soup

3 Tbsp. olive oil
1 onion
2 cloves of garlic
1 ½ c. green beads
1 c. kernels of corn
1 lb. acorn squash
1 jalapeno
14 oz. diced tomatoes
½ Tbsp. vinegar, white wine
½ c. vegetable stock
Pepper

Heat up the olive oil in a large skillet before adding garlic and an onion. Sauté up the garlic and the onion for several minutes until the onion is soft. Next you should add the jalapeno, green beans, and squash to the mixture and cook for about 5 minutes. Add all of the remaining ingredients and reduce the heat. Let the soup simmer for another 30 minutes and serve warm.

Gazpacho

2 c. yogurt
½ c. cilantro
1 bell pepper, red
4 tomatoes
1 onion
2 cucumbers
¼ vinegar, red wine
3 c. tomato juice
1 clove of garlic
2 tsp. pepper sauce
Pepper

Stir in the cilantro and the yogurt together and then set it aside. Cut up the half of the onion, one of the cucumbers, half a bell pepper, and two of the tomatoes and place them into a blender. Blend them all up before adding the remaining ingredients along with the yogurt and the mixed them up well. Dice up the rest of the onion, cucumber, bell pepper, and tomato and refrigerate them for 2 hours. Top your soup with a spoonful of the cilantro yogurt.

Chapter 4 – A Little Something Extra – Appetizers & Sides

Grilled Vegetables

½ c. vinegar, balsamic
1 ¼ c. yogurt
2 Tbsp. olive oil
3 sliced zucchini
2 garlic cloves
2 Tbsp. parsley
2 eggplants
1 onion
½ c. red pepper, roasted

Pour the vinegar into a sauce pan and let it simmer for a little bit before setting it aside and cool. Once it is cooled down you can mix it in with the parsley, garlic, oil, and yogurt. Divide this mixture up in half. After chopping up the onion, eggplant, and zucchini you will set them out a pan and brush with some of the yogurt mix, about half of it. Cook the vegetables for about 4 minutes. Place the veggies on a plate. Use the red peppers to sprinkle over the vegetables before adding the rest of the yogurt and serving.

Tomato and Zucchini Bake

4 c. zucchini
1 tsp. oil, vegetable
3 Tbsp. onion
¼ c. cheese, grated
2 c. tomatoes, sliced
Salt
Pepper

Preheat your oven to 375 degrees. While that is heating up you will need to wash the zucchini and then cut into thin slices. In a frying pan you should cook up the onion until tender and then add the zucchini and cook for another 5 minutes. Add the tomatoes to the onions and zucchini and cook for another 5 minutes. Put this mixture into a baking dish and add cheese. Bake up the mixture for another 20 minutes and then serve.

Potato Wedges

3 potatoes
3 Tbsp. olive oil
1 ½ tsp. paprika
1 ½ tsp. garlic
1 ½ tsp. chili powder
1 ½ powder of onion

Start by heating the oven up to 450 degrees. Scrub all excess dirt off the potatoes and then cut into wedges, 8 pieces. Next you should mix up the onion powder, chili powder, garlic powder, paprika, and oil and take the mixture and spread it onto the sides of the potato wedges. Place all of the wedges on one baking sheet and then bake for about 30 minutes

Squash Casserole

¼ c. egg
½ c. yellow onion
1 lb. squash
½ c. mayonnaise
½ c. bread crumbs
½ c. cheddar cheese
¼ tsp. black pepper
Salt

Preheat the oven to 350 degrees and while that is heating up you can slice the squash into thin slices and steam them up until they are soft. Next you should mix together pepper, salt, cheese, mayonnaise, onion, and egg before adding in the squash. Pour it all together in a casserole dish and top it off with the breadcrumbs. Put in the oven and bake for at least 30 minutes.

Sweet Potato Fries

1 sweet potatoes
½ tsp. cumin
½ tsp. paprika
1 Tbsp. olive oil
½ tsp. cayenne
½ tsp. oregano

Heat your oven to 400 degrees and then start preparing the food. Clean up your sweet potatoes before cutting them up lengthwise in half and continue to do this until they are small strips. Combine the seasonings, olive oil, and sweet potatoes in a plastic bag, close the bag and shake everything together until the fries or coated. Spread out the fries on a baking sheet before putting in the oven and baking for about 45 minutes. Make sure to rotate the fries every 15 minutes to cook them evenly.

Fiesta Lime Rice

1 ½ c. rice, long grain
¾ c. black beans
1 tomato
¾ c. corn
1 green onion
1 Tbsp. lime juice
4 Tbsp. cilantro
Salt

Find a bowl and combine the pre-cooked rice, lime juice, cilantro, green onion, tomato, beans, and corn together. Make sure they are mixed well together before adding in some salt and serving.

Chapter 5 –Italian Night – Pasta Dishes

Zesty Chicken Pasta

1 lb. chicken strips
12 oz. fettuccini pasta
1 Tbsp. vegetable oil
1 tsp. basil
16 oz. vegetable mix
½ c. parmesan cheese
½ c. salad dressing, Caesar
¼ c. black olives

Star by cooking up the pasta before adding the vegetables in during the last few minutes of cooking time. Let it boil until the vegetables are tender. You will then need to drain the water from the vegetables and pasta. Next you will need to heat up the oil before adding the chicken in. Sprinkle on some basil and cook the chicken until it is done which will be about 8 to 10 minutes. Add the vegetables and the pasta to the chicken before adding in the dressing. Cook until everything is warm. Before serving make sure to add the olives and cheese on top.

Squash Lasagna

2 c. marinara sauce
1 c. ricotta
3 c. spaghetti squash
8 tsp. parmesan cheese
6 oz. mozzarella
Red pepper

Start by roasting the spaghetti squash. You will need to cut the squash up in half and scoop the seeds out. Place the squash of the baking sheet and sprinkle on the pepper and the salt. Bake the squash for 60 minutes until the inside feels tender. Let it cool for about 10 minutes after removing the oven. Scrape out the flesh of the squash with a fork and measure out about 3 cups for this recipe. Warm up the oven to 375 degrees. Next take half the marinara sauce and spread it into a baking dish. Top it with the squash first, then the ricotta cheese and lastly with the mozzarella and the parmesan. Add the other half of the sauce before sprinkling on a little more cheese and pepper. Let it bake for another 20 minutes while covered with foil before removing the foil and adding on another 5 minutes.

One Pan Spaghetti

½ lb. ground beef
1 onion
3 ½ c. water
15 oz. tomato sauce
2 c. spaghetti, broken up
½ tsp. sugar
½ tsp. garlic powder
2 tsp. oregano
½ tsp. rosemary
4 oz. parmesan
Pepper

Start by browning up the onions and the beef in a skillet. Make sure to drain out the fat and grease before continuing. Next you will need to stir in the spices, tomato sauce and the water and make it all boil. Next you will add the spaghetti and then let it simmer for about 15 minutes; make sure to stir so the spaghetti does not stick. Once the cooking is done you can cover with cheese and serve.

Porcini Mushroom Pasta

¼ porcini mushrooms
1 tsp. butter
3 Tbsp. tomatoes, sun-dried
½ tsp. red onion
½ c. milk
Salt
White Pepper
½ lb. fettuccini
1 green onion
1 Tbsp. parmesan

Cover up the mushrooms with some hot water and let it stand there for about 10 minutes. Once the time is off you can drain the water off and cut up the mushrooms into small pieces. Melt the butter in a skillet and then add the red onion to sauté for around 1 minute. Next add in the tomatoes and mushrooms and sauté for another 3 minutes. After those ingredients have been cooked you can stir in the white pepper, salt, and milk and bring it all to a boil. Once it has reached a boil you may reduce the heat and let the whole mixture simmer for another 15 minutes. While that is simmering you are able to cook up the fettuccine until it is cooked, drain, and transfer it to a serving bowl. Pour all of the sauce onto the pasta and mix together. Top with the cheese and the scallions right before serving.

Pasta Ratatouille

6 c. water
3 Tbsp. vegetable oil
1 onion
6 garlic cloves
1 lb. pasta
3 zucchini
2 green peppers
1 eggplant
1 ½ tsp. salt
½ tsp. pepper
3 tomatoes
1 c. shredded Swiss cheese
2 tsp. basil

Bring some water to boil before adding the pasta and cooking it until it is tender. You will then need to drain the pasta and set it aside for later. Heat up some oil before adding the garlic and onion to it and sautéing both of them around 4 minutes. Next add in the eggplant, zucchini, and bell pepper for around 10 minutes of cooking and then add the seasonings and the tomatoes for another 3 minutes. Pour the vegetable mixture over the pasta and cover with some of the shredded cheese before serving.

Chapter 6 – The Main Event

Ginger Raspberry Chicken

1 ¼ lb. chicken breasts
2 Tbsp. olive oil
1 onion
Salt
Pepper
2 c. carrots
2 c. florets of broccoli
1 Tbsp. raspberry jam
1 T. vinegar, white wine
1 tsp. ginger
1 Tbsp. soy sauce
1 Tbsp. water

Start by seasoning the chicken breasts with some pepper and salt. Next you will need to heat up some oil for about 30 seconds before adding in the carrots and the onion and cook for about 5 more minutes. Next you need to add the chicken and broccoli and cook for an additional 8 minutes before moving the chicken and vegetables to a plate. Next you will need to combine the ginger, soy sauce, water, vinegar, and jam in the skillet and mix together for about 2 minutes. Marinate this with the chicken before stirring in with the vegetables. Cook until chicken is ready and then serve.

Quesadilla Pie

2 lb. rotisserie chicken
2 c. salsa, chunky
¼ c. sour cream
1 ½ c. cheddar cheese, shredded
1 c. spinach
3 tortillas

Preheat up the oven until it is 375 degrees. While the oven is heating up you will need to combine the sour cream, half the salsa, and the chicken in a bowl and spread another ½ c. of salsa onto the bottom of a baking dish. Next you will press in one of the tortillas into the baking dish and tap it off with about half the chicken and sprinkle with half the spinach and some cheese. Repeat this step but make sure to keep a little of the cheese for the end. On the final tortilla you can add the rest of the salsa and the leftover cheese. Cover the baking dish with foil and bake for about 20 minutes before removing the foil and baking another 5 minutes and then serve.

Southwestern Chicken

1 fillet of chicken breast
2 Tbsp. refried beans
1 Tbsp. cheese, Mexican blend
2 Tbsp. black beans
1 Tbsp. salsa
2 tortilla chips

Place the chicken breast on a plat and cook in the microwave for about 2 ½ minutes. Let this chicken stand for another 2 minutes before proceeding. Next you will need to cover the chicken with the cheese, black beans, and refried beans before microwaving for another 45 seconds. Top this chicken with the salsa and the tortilla chips.

Fish Tacos

2 lbs. fillet of cods
3 Tbsp. lime juice
½ onion
3 Tbsp. cilantro
1 tomato
1 tsp. olive oil
Cayenne pepper
Black pepper
Salt
2 c. cabbage, red
½ c. onion, green
¾ cup salsa
8 tortillas
¾ c. sour cream

Preheat up the oven to 350 degrees. Rinse off the fish and place on a dish to drain off the fat. Next you will need to mix together the salt, peppers, olive oil, cilantro, onion, tomato, and lime juice to use in covering the fillets. Cover this dish with some foil and bake for about 20 minutes. While that is baking you can mix together the onion and cabbage and the salsa and sour cream separately before combining together. Divide up the fish between the 8 tortillas and then add some of the cabbage mixture between them. Fold them over and then serve.

Shepherd's Pie

2 baking potatoes
½ c. milk
1 onion
2 Tbsp. flour
1 lb. ground beef
1 garlic clove
¼ c. beef broth
4 c. mixed vegetables, frozen
½ c. cheddar cheese
Pepper

Dice up the potatoes and then place them in a saucepan with just a little bit of water. Bring the water to a boil before reducing the heat and letting it simmer for about 15 minutes. Drain out these potatoes and then mash them up before adding the milk and setting aside. Next you can preheat up the oven to 375 degrees and while that is warming up you can add the garlic, onion and meat to a skillet and brown them up. Next stir in some flour and let it all cook for about a minute. After that time you can add in the broth and the vegetables and let cook for another 5 minutes. Spoon in the vegetables into a baking dish and spread the potato mix over the meat and vegetables. Sprinkle a little cheese on top. Put the baking dish in the oven and let bake for about 25 minutes.

Cheese, Turkey, and Pear Sandwich

1 slices of bread
2 tsp. mustard, Dijon
1 pear
¼ mozzarella cheese
2 slices smoked turkey
Pepper

Put the mustard on each piece of bread before placing a piece of turkey on each slice. Cut up the pear and arrange how you would like on the bread before adding a little bit of cheese to the sandwich. Broil the sandwich for several minutes until the cheese is melting. Cut the sandwich and serve.

Spicy Pork Tenderloin

¾ c. apple cider
2 Tbsp. syrup
¼ c. vinegar, apple cider
¼ tsp. paprika
1 tsp. black pepper
1 tsp. ginger
2 tsp. vegetable oil
12 oz. pork tenderloin
1 apple
1 sweet potato

Begin this recipe by preheating the oven up to 375 degrees and then combine the pepper, ginger, paprika, syrup, vinegar, and cider together in a bowl and then set it aside for a few minutes. Het some oil on the oven and then add the pork tenderloins on top. Cook this well until the pork is browned for about 12 minutes and then remove the pan from heat. Next place some sweet potatoes near the pork and more some of the apple cider mix over the pork. Cover this all and bake for about 20 minutes. Make sure the thickest part of pork has an internal temperature of 145. After the 20 minutes you will need to turn the sweet potatoes around and place the apples all around the pork. Bake this for about 10 more minutes until the pork reaches 170 degrees. Remove the sweet potatoes, apples, and pork from the pan and let it stand and cool. As that cools you will need to reduce apple cider a little and then slice up the pork. Serve the pork along with the apples and sweet potatoes and pour cider over everything.

Pita Pizza

2 pieces pita bread
¼ c. tomato sauce
1/3 c. mozzarella cheese
Any veggies

Turn on the oven to about 350 degrees. While this is heating up you should split the bread in half and add in the tomato sauce, any toppings that you choose, and the cheese. Wrap up each piece of bread in some foil and cook for about 7 to 10 minutes.

Southwest Tortilla Bake

8 tortillas
1 c. cheese, Monterey Jack
1 c. corn
2 onions
3 eggs
1 c. pinto beans
4 oz. green chilies
½ tsp. chili powder
1 c. milk
1 tomato
Salsa

Start by heating up the oven to 350 degrees. Arrange 5 halves of the tortilla to the bottom of a baking pan and then cover them with about 1/3 c. of the beans, corn, and cheese before springing about half the onions on top of that. Add another 5 halves on top of that and do another 1/3 c. cheese along with the rest of the onions, beans, and corn before adding the final 5 halves of the tortilla over everything. After that is done you can add the chili powder, milk and eggs together and mix before stirring the green chilies in. Pour this mixture on top of the tortillas and top with the remaining cheese and the tomato slices. Bake it all for around 50 minutes and let it stand for another 10 minutes before serving.

West and East Stir-fry

1 Tbsp. ginger
1 garlic clove
4 oz. pork loin
1 carrot
2 bell peppers
1 ½ c. onions, sliced
1 c. celery
2 Tbsp. soy sauce
½ c. water, cold
2 tsp. cornstarch
4 c. rice, cooked
6 oz. dried plums

Start out by putting a skillet over high heat before adding the garlic and the ginger and heating it for about 1 minute. Add the pork and cook for another two minutes before adding the celery and peppers to the mix and cooking an additional 4 minutes. Add in the plums and cook until heated through. At the same time combine the cornstarch and the soy sauce and mix together before adding this mixture in and stirring another two minutes. Divide out the rice and top with the stir-fry ingredients before serving.

Cheeseburgers

1 lb. beef
2 Tbsp. oats
4 hamburger buns
½ tsp. steak seasoning
4 slices cheese
Any toppings

Start by placing the oats in a plastic bag and use a rolling pin to crush the oats up. Next you will need to combine the steak seasoning, oats, and ground beef together before shaping into 4 patties. Place the patties on the grill and let them cook to your preferred liking. While those are cooking you can put any toppings that you like, lettuce, tomatoes, ketchup, mustard, on the buns and then top with the hamburger.

Chapter 7 –Decadent Desserts

Oat Nut Blackberry Crumble

2 Tbsp. sugar
2 c. blackberries
1 Tbsp. cornstarch
½ c. oats
½ tsp. lemon juice
¼ c. brown sugar
½ tsp. cinnamon
1/3 cup flour
1 Tbsp. butter
¼ c. hazelnuts
Salt

Start by preheating the oven up to 350 degrees. In a bowl combine the cornstarch and the sugar together before adding in the lemon juice and the berries. Pour all of this into a baking dish. Next you will need another bowl in order to mix together the salt, cinnamon, brown sugar, flour and oats. Add the butter in but make sure to cut into smaller pieces for easier mixing. Lastly stir in the hazelnuts. Spread this topping over your berry mixture and then place in the oven. This will need to bake for about 30 minutes.

Pumpkin Pie

1 c. ginger snaps
½ c. egg whites
16 oz. pumpkin, canned
½ c. sugar
12 oz. evaporated milk
2 tsp. pumpkin spice

Preheat up the oven to 350 degrees before grinding up the ginger snaps in a blender. Take the cookies and line a baking pan evenly. Next you will need to mix the egg whites, sugar, pumpkin, evaporated milk, and the pumpkin spice together in a bowl before pour into the crust you already have. Bake the pie for about 45 minutes and then place it in the refrigerator to set.

Frozen Yogurt

1 c. strawberries
1 c. raspberries
1 c. blueberries
1 Tbsp. sugar
3 Tbsp. orange juice
1 tsp. orange zest
1 pint yogurt.

Combine the strawberries, raspberries, and blueberries together with the sugar in a bowl. Use a grater to remove the orange zest that you need and add that to all the berries. Slice the orange and squeeze it for the required orange juice and combine everything together. Let it all chill overnight. When ready to serve place some yogurt in each bowl and top with the berries.

Chocolate Oatmeal Cookies

2 c. oats
½ c. flour, all purpose
½ c. flour, pastry
½ tsp. baking soda
1 tsp. cinnamon
Salt
½ c. tahini
2/3 cup sugar
4 Tbsp. butter
2/3 cup brown sugar
1 egg
1 Tbsp. vanilla
1 egg white
1 c. chocolate chips
½ c. walnuts

Preheat the oven to 350 degrees. While that is happening line several baking sheets with liners. Next you should combine the salt, baking soda, cinnamon, both flours, and the oats together in a bowl. Then you will need to beat in the butter and the tahini in until it is a paste and add both the sugars until the mixture is a little grainy. Next add in the vanilla, egg white, and vanilla before stirring in the oat mixture and then the walnuts and chocolate chips. Take the batter and roll about a tablespoon into a ball and put on the baking sheet; do this until the sheet is full and then place in the oven. Let them bake for 16 minutes. Let them cool for a few minutes before transferring off the pan to finish cooling. Enjoy right away or store them for later.

Oatmeal Streusel with Pears and Cranberry

¾ c. oats
1 c. brown sugar
½ tsp. cinnamon
1 Tbsp. butter
¼ tsp. nutmeg
3 c. pears
2 ½ Tbsp. cornstarch
2 c. cranberries
Pie crust

Preheat the oven to about 350 degrees and then start preparing the streusel by combining half the brown sugar, the oats, cinnamon, and nutmeg before adding in the butter until it looks like coarse meal. Next you will need to prepare the filling by combining the corn starch, rest of brown sugar, cranberries, and pears and mixing together. Spoon this mixture into the pastry and then sprinkle on the streusel. Bake this for about 1 hour and then let cool for another hour before serving.

Chocolate Pudding

3 Tbsp. cornstarch
2 Tbsp. sugar
2 Tbsp. cocoa powder
2 c. milk
1/3 c. chocolate chips
Salt
½ tsp. vanilla

Mix together the salt, sugar, cocoa powder, and cornstarch together in a bowl and then add in the milk. Heat this mixture on the stove until it is beginning to thicken and bubble. Once this happens you can take it away from the heat and add in the vanilla and the chocolate chips. Stir until the pudding is smooth. Serve right away or set in the refrigerator to chill.

Pear and Strawberry Trifle

2 pears
2 Tbsp. lemon juice
½ tsp. extract of almond
2 Tbsp. orange juice
2 c. strawberries
2 Tbsp. honey
3 c. yogurt, lemon flavor
Half of an angel food cake

Start by setting the pears in the almond extract, strawberries, and lemon juice before combining it with the honey and orange juice and mixing it together. You will then need to start layering the baking pan starting with some of the cake, a third of the orange juice mixture you just made, a cup of the lemon yogurt, some pears, and some strawberries. Repeat this step a second time. Finally you should layer on the rest of the cake and sprinkle with any orange juice left over along with the yogurt. Cover and let it cool for a couple hours before you serve.

Apple Cranberry Risotto

½ c. cranberries, dried
1 stick of cinnamon
Salt
3 ½ c. milk
1 apple, golden delicious
½ c. rice, Arborio
2 Tbsp. brown sugar
1 ½ c. apple cider
1 Tbsp. butter

Start by covering up the cranberries with the water and then let them set for up to 30 minutes in order to plump up. Heat up the salt, cinnamon stick, and milk in a microwave or on the stove until hot but it is not boiling and set it to the side to steep. Heat some butter up and then add the apple to cook for 2 minutes before adding the rice and cooking another 30 seconds. Next add ¾ c. apple cider to the mix and stir it for about 2 minutes before adding in the sugar. When that is all cooked you can mix in the milk and cinnamon to this mixture and let it absorb for 3 more minutes. Add in the remaining milk slowly until the rice feels tender and the dish is creamy. Remove from heat and throw out any cinnamon still left. Drain the cranberries from the water and stir it into the risotto with a little vanilla. Let it cool for about 10 minutes and then serve.

www.ingramcontent.com/pod-product-compliance
Lightning Source LLC
Chambersburg PA
CBHW080447290526
45791CB00008BA/2636